Dr. Salvatore G. Matheson

HEALTHY HOLIDAYS

Preventing Heart Attacks And Maintaining Heart Health

Contents

1.

2.

3.

4.

5.

6.

7.

8.

9.

Introduction

Winter Vacations And Heart Attack Deaths

The winter holidays can be dangerous, according to a study, as more individuals die from heart attacks during the last week of December than at any other time of the year. While being aware of the indications of a heart attack and taking steps to minimize your risk is important throughout the year, the American Heart Association notes that it is especially crucial during the holiday season.

According to a study published in Circulation, the American Heart Association's flagship publication, more cardiac deaths occur in the United States on December 25 than any other day of the year, followed by December 26 and January 1. According to a British Medical Journal study that looked at more than 16 years of data on heart attacks in Sweden, there was a 15% overall rise in heart attacks during the winter holidays, with heart attacks climbing 37% on December 24 (Christmas Eve).

One of the most essential aspects could be that people fail to recognize important warning signals of a heart attack or stroke. The American Heart Association recommends recognizing symptoms early and dialing 9-1-1 for assistance. The earlier medical care is started, the better the odds of survival and avoiding heart damage.

It is critical to be aware of the signs and symptoms of a heart attack over the holiday season and to take action if you or someone you know has any of the following symptoms:

-Discomfort or pain in the chest
    -Pain in an arm, neck, or jaw
    -Breathing difficulty
    -Vomiting or nausea
    - Perspiring
    -Feeling dizzy

In addition to being aware of heart attack symptoms, it is critical to maintain a healthy lifestyle throughout the holidays and throughout the year. This includes eating a well-balanced diet, exercising on a regular basis, maintaining a healthy weight, not smoking, and getting adequate rest. You can help ensure a better and happier holiday season for yourself and your loved ones by being aware of the signs of a heart attack and adopting preventive actions.

What Exactly Is A Heart Attack?

A heart attack, also known as a myocardial infarction, happens when blood supply to a portion of the heart is interrupted, resulting in damage to the heart muscle. It is a life-threatening medical emergency that requires immediate treatment to prevent cardiac damage and death. The following are frequent symptoms of a heart attack:

-Chest discomfort: This might feel like pressure, tightness, heaviness, squeezing, or pain in the chest, and it can linger for several minutes or come and go.

-Pain or discomfort in other upper body areas: Symptoms may include pain or discomfort in one or both arms, the back, neck, jaw, or stomach.

-Shortness of breath: This can occur with or without chest tightness and may indicate a heart attack.

Other symptoms: These include cold sweat, weariness, heartburn or indigestion, dizziness, nausea, and pain or discomfort in the jaw, neck, or back.

It's crucial to remember that men and women experience different heart attack symptoms, with women more likely to experience atypical symptoms such as extreme exhaustion, shortness of breath, and nausea or vomiting. A heart attack can occur without any obvious symptoms in rare situations, a condition known as a "silent" heart attack, which is more common in diabetics.

If you or someone else is suffering symptoms of a heart attack, get medical attention immediately. It is critical to contact 911 or emergency medical services as soon as possible in order to receive the appropriate treatment. Medication, surgical procedures, and lifestyle modifications may be used to treat a heart attack and prevent repeat episodes. Maintaining a nutritious diet, getting regular exercise, and avoiding smoking are all essential factors in preventing heart disease and lowering the risk of having a heart attack.

Recognizing heart attack signs and receiving urgent medical attention can save lives. Understanding the warning symptoms and risk factors, as well as living a heart-healthy lifestyle, are critical steps in preventing heart disease and lowering the odds of having a heart attack.

Symptoms of a minor heart attack

A tiny heart attack, also known as a silent heart attack, is a form of heart attack that causes no acute symptoms and is sometimes misdiagnosed as indigestion or muscle soreness. Symptoms of a heart attack include pressure, tightness, pain, squeezing, or aching in the chest; pain that spreads to the arms, neck, jaw, or back; a feeling of crushing or heaviness in the chest; nausea and sometimes vomiting; feeling clammy and sweaty; shortness of breath; feeling lightheaded or dizzy; and, in some cases, no symptoms at all. To avoid complications and death, it is critical to recognize the early signs of a heart attack and seek immediate medical assistance. If you or someone you know is having heart attack symptoms, dial 911 or your local emergency number right away.

It's important to remember that men and women experience different heart attack symptoms, with women being more likely to encounter unusual symptoms such as acute tiredness, shortness of breath, nausea, or vomiting. In rare cases, a heart attack can occur without any evident symptoms, a condition known as a "silent" heart attack, which is more common in diabetics.

If you or someone else is experiencing heart attack symptoms, seek medical attention right away. It is vital to call 911 or emergency medical services as soon as possible in order to receive proper care. Medication, surgical procedures, and lifestyle changes may be utilized to treat a heart attack and prevent it from happening again. A balanced diet, regular exercise, and quitting smoking are all important factors in preventing heart disease and lowering the chance of having a heart attack.

Recognizing the symptoms of a heart attack and seeking immediate medical assistance can save lives. Understanding the warning signs and risk factors, as well as leading a heart-healthy lifestyle, are important measures in preventing heart disease and lowering the chances of having a heart attack.

Heart Attack Causes And Risk Factors

A heart attack, also known as a myocardial infarction, happens when blood supply to a portion of the heart is interrupted, resulting in damage to the heart muscle. It is a life-threatening medical emergency that requires immediate treatment to prevent cardiac damage and death. Heart attacks are most commonly caused by constriction and blockage of the coronary arteries, which reduce blood flow to the heart. Some of the most important risk factors for a heart attack are:

1. Age: Men over the age of 45 and women over the age of 55 are more likely to have a heart attack than younger people.

2. Family history: A close family relative with a history of heart disease at a young age increases the risk of having a heart attack.

3. High LDL cholesterol (the "bad" cholesterol) and triglyceride levels: High levels of LDL cholesterol (the "bad" cholesterol) and triglycerides can raise the risk of heart attack.

4. High blood pressure: High blood pressure can damage arteries leading to the heart over time, and high blood pressure that co-occurs with other illnesses such as obesity, high cholesterol, or diabetes raises the risk even more.

5. Smoking: Tobacco use raises the risk of heart attack and impairs the efficacy of other treatments.

6. Obesity: Obesity raises the risk of heart attacks and other cardiovascular disorders, particularly central obesity.

7. Diabetes: High blood glucose levels raise the risk of having a heart attack or having a stroke.

8. Unhealthy diet: A diet heavy in processed foods, trans fats, and salt raises the risk of heart attack.

9. Physical inactivity: A sedentary lifestyle and a lack of exercise can contribute to the development of heart disease.

10. Stress: Emotional stress, such as severe rage, may raise the risk of having a heart attack.

11. Illegal drug use: Cocaine and amphetamines can cause coronary artery spasms, which can lead to a heart attack.

Recognizing and controlling these risk factors through healthy lifestyle choices, medical measures, and, in some situations, emergency treatment are all part of preventing heart attacks. Individuals can take proactive efforts to lower their risk and maintain a healthy heart by learning the causes and risk factors for heart attacks.

Lifestyle Changes And Healthy Habits As Preventive Measures

Heart disease is the largest cause of mortality worldwide, although it is preventable in many situations by lifestyle modifications and healthy practices. A healthy lifestyle can lower the risk of heart disease and heart attack by up to 80%. Here are some preventative practices that may be useful:

1. Quit smoking: Smoking is a major risk factor for cardiovascular disease and heart attack. One of the most significant steps you can take to improve your heart health is to quit smoking.

2. Maintain a healthy weight: Being overweight or obese increases your chances of developing heart disease and other health issues. Maintaining a healthy weight through a well-balanced diet and regular exercise can help lower your risk of heart disease.

3. Exercise regularly: Regular physical activity can help minimize your risk of heart disease and heart attack. Strive for 2.5 hours per week of moderate-intensity exercise, such as brisk walking, cycling, or swimming

4. Maintain a healthy diet: Eating a nutritious diet will help lower your risk of heart disease and stroke. Consume a wide range of fruits and vegetables, whole grains, lean proteins, and healthy fats. Consume fewer processed meals, saturated and trans fats, and added sweets.

5. Manage stress: Chronic stress has been linked to an increased risk of heart disease and heart attack. Get healthful stress-relieving activities such as exercise, meditation, or spending time with loved ones.

6. Get enough sleep: Sleep deprivation, both in terms of quality and length, can raise the risk of heart disease and heart attack. Work towards 7-8 hours of sleep for every night and stick to a consistent sleep schedule.

7. Limit alcohol consumption: Excessive alcohol use might raise blood pressure and contribute to heart disease. Limit your alcohol consumption to one drink per day for ladies and two drinks per day for men.

8. Practice hands-only CPR: Chronic illnesses such as high blood pressure, high cholesterol, and diabetes can all raise the risk of heart disease and heart attack. Manage these disorders with medicine, lifestyle adjustments, and regular check-ups in collaboration with your healthcare professional.

Individuals can dramatically minimize their risk of heart disease and heart attack by adopting these healthy habits. It is crucial to remember that these lifestyle modifications do not demand a one-time commitment or effort. Small changes can have a major impact on heart health and general well-being.

Heart Attack Medications And Treatment

Treatment for a heart attack is critical to preventing further heart muscle damage and restoring blood flow. The precise treatment depends on whether the blood flow is partially or completely blocked. Heart attack medications and therapies include:

1. Antiplatelet medicines: Such as aspirin, clopidogrel (Plavix), prasugrel (Effient), and ticagrelor (Brilinta), are used to minimize blood clotting and keep a heart attack from worsening.

2. Thrombolytic therapy: the use of clot-busting medicines to dissolve blood clots in the arteries of the heart.

3. Anticoagulants (blood thinners): These drugs, such as heparin or warfarin, help prevent blood clot formation.

4. Nitroglycerin: This drug helps to reduce chest pain by widening blood vessels and increasing blood flow to the heart.

5. Beta blockers: These medications reduce blood pressure and the burden on the heart by slowing the heart rate and force of contraction.

6. ACE Inhibitors: These blood pressure medications lower blood pressure and minimize heart stress.

7. Discomfort relievers: Medications such as morphine are used to treat chest discomfort that does not respond to nitroglycerin.

8. Statins: These pharmaceuticals, often known as cholesterol-lowering medications, help lower harmful cholesterol levels.

Surgical and other procedures, in addition to drugs, may be required to unblock a blocked artery and restore blood flow. These methods are as follows:

1. Coronary angioplasty and stenting: During this procedure, a specialist inserts a balloon to expand the blocked artery and a stent to keep it open.

2. Percutaneous coronary intervention (PCI): A catheter is used to unblock a blocked artery in this minimally invasive treatment.

If you have signs of a heart attack, get immediate medical assistance because early treatment can greatly improve results and reduce the chance of long-term consequences.

The Role Of Emergency Medical Services (EMS) In The Response To A Heart Attack

The role of emergency medical services (EMS) in responding to out-of-hospital cardiac arrests and suspected heart attacks is crucial. The EMS system is intended to provide prehospital emergency medical care, and its performance can have a substantial impact on patient outcomes. Several critical components of the EMS response to cardiac crises deserve special attention:

1. Personnel and Oversight: The EMS system employs a diverse group of professionals who perform important services such as responding to 911 emergency calls, dispatching medical personnel, triage, and treatment. The general structure, service organization, and capabilities of EMS systems can all have a significant impact on the quality and speed of care provided to those having cardiac crises.

2. Response Times and Bystander CPR: In the context of cardiac crises, EMS response times are critical, as delays can have a major impact on patient outcomes. Efforts to improve the timeliness and quality of care offered to people in communities across the United

States include efforts to encourage bystander CPR and early defibrillation procedures.

3. Integration with Health Services: In the future, EMS is expected to be fully integrated with other health care providers, as well as public health and public safety authorities. EMS will be able to identify and modify sickness and injury risks, provide acute illness and injury care and follow-up, and contribute to the treatment of chronic conditions and community health monitoring as a result of this integration.

4. Research and development: The EMS system is always evolving, especially in the context of greater changes in the health care system. As a result, continual research and development are required to reinforce the infrastructure and improve the science of EMS, ultimately improving community health.

5. Quality of Care and Patient Outcomes: The usage of emergency medical services (EMS) in acute myocardial infarction and other cardiac events has a direct impact on the patient's overall care and subsequent quality of care. EMS systems are always changing to handle the broad collection of research studies and initiatives aimed at minimizing the burden of cardiac events and other emergencies that fall under their purview of treatment.

Finally, EMS plays a diverse and critical role in responding to cardiac events such as out-of-hospital cardiac arrests and suspected heart attacks. Several elements influence the system's performance, including response times, integration with health services, and continuing research and development activities. EMS contributes considerably to the well-being and outcomes of patients undergoing cardiac emergencies by constantly seeking to enhance the speed and quality of care.

Cpr With Your Hands: A Lifesaving Skill For Everyone

Hands-only CPR is a simplified variant of standard CPR that anyone, regardless of training level, may perform. It is as simple as dialing 911 and starting chest compressions. Hands-only CPR is a lifesaving skill that can increase a person's odds of survival after a cardiac arrest by doubling or tripling their chances.

Traditional CPR entails a combination of chest compressions and rescue breaths, which can be daunting for some people and may necessitate additional training. Hands-only CPR, on the other hand, is a simpler approach that is rapid and easy to master. It is advised to use it on adults who have collapsed and are unresponsive.

Bystanders who witness a cardiac arrest should call 911 immediately and begin hands-only CPR until emergency medical personnel arrive, according to the American Heart Association (AHA) [2]. Individuals who are not trained in CPR should nevertheless attempt hands-only CPR if they see a cardiac arrest, as any attempt at CPR is preferable to none.

Hands-only CPR requires conducting chest compressions at a rate of 100–120 beats per minute, which is around the same speed as the

Bee Gees' song "Stayin' Alive." Push strongly and quickly in the center of the chest, allowing the chest to fully recoil between compressions.

Everyone should learn hands-only CPR since cardiac arrest can happen to anybody, anywhere, at any time. Individuals who learn hands-only CPR can be prepared to respond in an emergency and perhaps save a life. The American Heart Association (AHA) provides a range of resources and training programs to help people learn hands-only CPR, including online courses, in-person training, and instructional films.

Finally, hands-only CPR is a simple and effective technique that anyone, regardless of their training level, may practice. It is as simple as dialing 911 and starting chest compressions. Individuals who learn hands-only CPR can be prepared to respond in an emergency and perhaps save a life. The American Heart Association provides a number of materials and training programs to help people learn hands-only CPR, which is a lifesaving skill that everyone should know.

Family Health History And The Risk Of Heart Disease

The health history of one's family is important in determining one's risk of acquiring heart disease. A positive family history of early heart disease is a known risk factor for heart disease, according to research, underscoring the necessity of describing its incidence and influence on cardiovascular health. You are more likely to acquire heart disease if you have a family history of the condition. Heart disease and related diseases, such as high blood pressure and excessive cholesterol, can run in families.

Knowing your family's health history is important since it can help you determine your own risk of heart disease. In your family health history evaluation, you should include your parents, siblings, children, grandparents, aunts, uncles, nieces, and nephews. It's also vital to keep track of which relatives have had heart illness, related disorders, or operations, as well as the age at which they were diagnosed or treated and the age and cause of death of relatives who have died.

A family health history can assist healthcare providers in identifying individuals who are at a higher risk of developing heart disease and recommending suitable preventive or treatment measures. If you have been diagnosed with heart disease or a related ailment, it is critical to inform your family members so that they can estimate their risk and take the required precautions.

Having a family member with heart disease at a young age (age 50 or under) can be a symptom of a hereditary illness that produces excessive cholesterol in some circumstances. As a result, gathering and sharing family health history information is critical for identifying potential genetic variables that may contribute to the risk of heart disease.

You can collaborate with your healthcare practitioner to establish a personalized plan for avoiding or managing heart disease by learning and sharing your family's health history. This could involve changes to one's lifestyle, regular health exams, and, in certain situations, genetic testing or counseling.

Finally, family health history is an important tool for determining an individual's risk of heart disease. Individuals can take proactive steps to prevent heart disease and its effects by collecting and sharing this information with healthcare providers. It is important that you update your family health history on a regular basis and notify your doctor of any new diagnoses, diseases, or operations in your family. If you are concerned about your personal or family history of heart disease, speak with your healthcare practitioner for personalized   advice   and   care.

What Should I Do To Recover From A Heart Attack?

Your heart can be injured if you've had a heart attack. This may interfere with your heart's rhythm and capacity to pump blood to the rest of your body. You could also be at risk for another heart attack or other diseases like stroke, renal problems, and peripheral arterial disease (PAD).

Following a heart attack, you can reduce your odds of experiencing future health problems by taking the following steps:

1. Physical activity: Discuss with your health care provider what you do every day in your life and at work. After a heart attack, your doctor may advise you to reduce your employment, travel, and sexual activity for a period of time.

2. Lifestyle changes: In addition to taking prescription medications, eating a healthy diet, increasing physical activity, stopping smoking, and managing stress can help improve your heart health and quality of life. In order to help you make these lifestyle changes, talk to your doctor about enrolling in a cardiac rehabilitation program.

3. Cardiac rehabilitation: a vital program for anyone recuperating from a heart attack, heart failure, or other heart disease that necessitated surgery or medical care. Cardiac rehabilitation is a monitored therapy that involves

- Physical exercise

- Education on healthy living, including good food, taking prescribed medications, and methods to help you quit smoking

- Counseling to alleviate stress and improve mental health

Your health care team, fitness and nutrition specialists, physical therapists, and counselors or mental health professionals may all assist you with cardiac rehab.

Conclusion

Tips for a Heart-Healthy Holiday Season

The Christmas season is a time for celebration, but it can also be a time for overindulgence and unhealthy habits that can harm your heart. However, by following a few basic guidelines, it is feasible to enjoy the holiday season while leading a heart-healthy lifestyle. Here are some heart-healthy holiday preparation tips:

1. Be aware of portion sizes: It's easy to overeat during the holidays, but being aware of portion proportions can help prevent overeating. To help reduce portion sizes, use smaller dishes, take smaller servings, and appreciate each bite.

2. Maintain a regular physical exercise schedule: Regular physical activity is vital for heart health, and the Christmas season is no exception. Incorporate physical activity into your holiday routine by going for a stroll after meals or signing up for holiday-themed exercise courses.

3. Choose nutritious foods: While many holiday foods are heavy in calories, fat, and sugar, there are many healthier alternatives. Choose fruits and vegetables, whole grains, lean meats, and healthy fats over processed and high-fat items.

4. Stay hydrated: Drinking plenty of water will help prevent overeating and dehydration, both of which can harm your heart. Aim for at least eight glasses of water every day, and keep sugary and alcoholic beverages to a minimum.

5. Get enough sleep: Sleep deprivation raises the risk of heart disease and other health concerns. To increase sleep quality, aim for seven to eight hours of sleep per night and maintain a consistent sleep regimen.

6. Manage stress: The holiday season can be stressful, but stress can harm your heart. Get healthful stress-relieving activities such as exercise, meditation, or passing time with loved ones.

7. Limit alcohol consumption: Excessive alcohol use might raise blood pressure and contribute to heart disease. Limit your alcohol consumption to one drink per day for ladies and two drinks per day for men.

8. Practice hands-only CPR: Knowing how to perform hands-only CPR can save a life throughout the holiday season. The American Heart Association provides tools and training programs to those interested in learning hands-only CPR.

Individuals can enjoy the Christmas season while maintaining a healthy lifestyle by following these heart-friendly tips. It's crucial to remember that even minor changes can have a major impact on heart health and general well-being. Please consult the sources listed for more information.

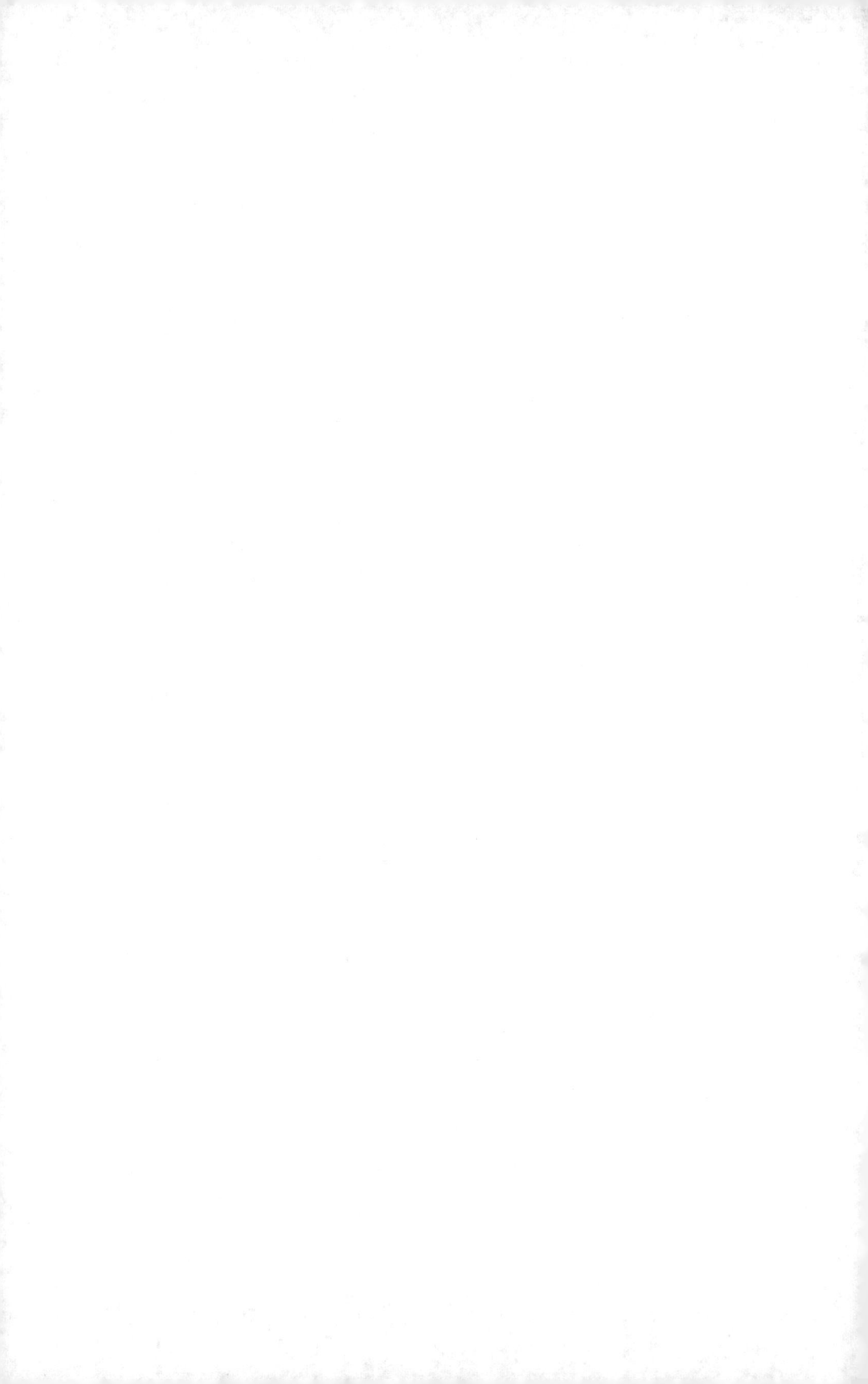